# HOW TO EXPLAIN PERIODS TO GIRLS

An Ultimate Guide to Talking To Your

Daughter About Her Periods

# Morin Gravelle

# INTRODUCTION

## *Overview of Periods and Why It Is Important To Explain Them to Girls*

The beginning of menstruation marks an important milestone in the life of a girl. It signifies the transition from childhood to womanhood and marks the beginning of a woman's reproductive years. As such, it is important to explain periods and other related facts to girls to help them prepare and understand their menstrual cycle, its effects on their bodies, their emotional health, and society's role in the experience.

## *The Age of Menarche*

The age of menarche is the onset of a female's first menstrual period. It typically occurs around age 12 but can occur anywhere from 8 to 16 years of age. It marks the beginning of a girl's reproductive life and the end of her childhood. This age represents a crucial point in a female's physical, psychological, and social development.

The age of menarche is of utmost importance in terms of development as it is a time of increased physical, emotional, and intellectual maturity. A female enters into a more advanced stage of maturity than when she was a child, and this is often combined with increased levels of anxiety and self-doubt. The hormonal changes associated with entering into the menstrual cycle can lead to alterations in behavior and mood.

The physiological aspect of the age of menarche is also very important, as it is a signal that a female has reached sexual maturity. The biological implications of this event are related to the woman's fertility, as menarche marks the beginning of potentially being able to conceive. It is also a sign of good health, given that the female has reached a suitable age to start ovulating.

The psychological aspect is also very significant at this time, as a young female is experiencing several new and unfamiliar emotions. The onset of menstruation leads to a sense of personal power and autonomy as her body begins to produce its hormones. However, it can also bring about a sense of uncertainty and apprehension, as she may feel that she is entering an unknown world.

The social aspect of menarche is also key, as it typically marks the transition from childhood to adulthood. A female is no longer considered a child and instead is treated as an adult among her peers and in society in general. It is an event that symbolizes a girl's ability to take on more responsibilities, and it can be a source of both pride and anxiety.

The age of menarche is an essential event in a woman's life and should never be seen as trivial. It is both a physical and psychological transformation and a time of great emotional and social development. It marks the end of childhood and the beginning of a woman's journey into adulthood.

The term "menarche" refers to the onset of a woman's first menstrual period. It usually occurs around the age of 12 in developed countries, but this age can vary depending on various factors such as race, genetics, and nutrition. The average age for menarche in the United States is 12.8 years old.

Throughout history, menarche has been viewed in a variety of ways. In some cultures, menarche is seen as a cause for celebration, with gifts and sometimes even formal ceremonies to mark the occasion. In others, it may be viewed with fear or as a punishment for some transgression.

What is most important, however, is what the event of menarche means to the individual woman. In terms of physical transformation, menarche signifies the beginning of the reproductive phase of a woman's life. Moreover, it is a sign that her body has reached the age of maturity and is now capable of bearing children. This new ability can be both exciting and frightening as women adjust to their new independence and greater responsibility.

On the psychological level, menarche can be viewed as a period of growth and change. It is a sign that a woman is no longer a girl, but has become a young adult. With this newfound maturity often come newfound confidence and self-awareness, as well as increased independence and responsibility.

At this age, social attitudes and norms also begin to take on greater importance. As a woman matures, she begins to focus on how she is seen regarding gender roles and sexual norms. She also begins to think about romantic relationships and what type of relationships she wants for her future.

The significance of menarche should not be underestimated. It is a life-altering experience that can shape a woman's future and sense of self. It is a time for both celebration and contemplation and should be embraced as an important milestone in a woman's journey toward maturity.

## *Periods and Cycle*

The menstrual cycle is the recurrence of bleeding from the vagina that occurs as part of the reproductive process in females. The duration of a menstrual cycle varies from woman to woman but often occurs over 28 days. Generally, the average time between periods is between 21 and 35 days. During this time, hormones in the body are preparing the uterus for childbirth, by building up a lining of blood and tissue.

At the end of the cycle, the body releases an egg and the lining of the uterus is shed in a process called menstruation. Most women experience bleeding for three to five days, although the length of time can vary significantly and can be longer in some cases. The color of the bloodshed during periods is usually red but also can have hints of brown or black.

***What Girls Should Know About Periods***

It is important to educate girls about the menstrual cycle to ensure that they understand the changes their bodies undergo and how to take care of themselves throughout this process. Girls should be guided to:

1. Learn about the anatomy of female reproductive organs, the difference between the menstruation cycle and fertile window, and why it is important to track the menstrual cycle.

2. Understand the emotional changes that may accompany the menstrual cycle.

3. Learn about different methods of contraception, and how to use them as well as the potential side effects of using hormonal contraception.

4. Learn about the associated symptoms that might accompany the menstrual cycle, such as cramps, headaches, and mood swings, and how to manage them.

5. Know when to seek medical advice and be aware of the mental health implications of pre-menstrual syndrome (P.M.S.) and other common issues.

## *Why Is It Important To Explain Periods to Girls*

The onset of periods is a time of great physical and emotional change for girls, which can be anxiety-triggering and may lead to feelings of isolation if not addressed. It is therefore important to equip girls with accurate knowledge about periods and the associated physical and emotional changes. Providing accurate information not only gives girls the confidence to manage the physical and psychological symptoms of their menstrual cycle, but it also helps to break the stigma and taboos that are still prevalent in many societies when it comes to discussing periods.

Through education and open dialogue, girls can learn how to look after themselves both physically and emotionally during this time and make sure they are adequately prepared for their transition into womanhood. Moreover, education about periods also helps to teach girls about consent, healthy relationships, and reproductive health. Explaining periods to girls is essential for them to make well-informed decisions about their health and live with dignity and autonomy.

# CHAPTER 1

## *Preparing Yourself and Your Girls for the Conversations*

Periods are a normal part of life, yet it can still be an uncomfortable topic for girls and women to talk about or ask questions about. Considering the taboos and stereotypes that remain around periods and the lack of knowledge surrounding female anatomy, it is understandable why women and young girls may feel uneasy about discussing the topic. But talking about periods can be beneficial for many reasons, such as improving girls' understanding of their bodies and how to care for themselves, equipping them with the knowledge and confidence to handle sensitive situations, and empowering them to feel comfortable with a topic that often gets swept under the rug. Preparing yourself and girls for conversations on periods is an important step in breaking the stigma and misinformation surrounding menstruation.

We'll cover the importance of talking about periods, the best techniques for preparing yourself and girls for conversations on periods, and helpful talking points that may arise.

<u>**Importance of Talking About Periods**</u>

The importance of talking about periods cannot be overstated. Periods can be confusing and overwhelming experiences, especially for young girls who are just beginning to menstruate. Having a friendly and open conversation can help clear up any confusion, as well as help girls feel more informed and confident. Talking about periods can also help break the stigma surrounding them and empower young girls to ask questions and assert their rights if needed.

In addition, talking about periods can assist in improving the overall health and well-being of girls and women. This includes providing the necessary information to take care of themselves during their cycles, from nutrition to menstrual product options. Having the necessary knowledge can help girls and women effectively manage their periods and reduce any pain or discomfort associated with them.

## Best Practices for Preparing Yourself

When preparing yourself for a conversation about periods with girls, it is important to be as prepared as possible. Researching menstrual health and proper menstrual hygiene can help you feel informed and confident when speaking to girls about their bodies. Starting with basic anatomy and physiology can also be helpful, as many girls may not be familiar with the terms or bodily functions associated with periods. This can help them better understand the topic and feel more comfortable asking questions.

In addition to the research, take time to consider the conversation as a whole. Think about your audience and any potential questions they may have. Brainstorm potential talking points relevant to their age and experience. Practice your conversation beforehand to ensure that you can speak confidently and answer any questions that come up.

Best Practices for Preparing Girls

When preparing girls for a conversation on periods, it is important to respect their age and level of knowledge. This can include providing them with an introduction to the topic using helpful resources or discussing their experiences in a comfortable, non-judgmental space. Use age-appropriate language and examples so that girls can better understand the topics discussed.

Encourage girls to ask questions and express their opinions about the topic. This can help them feel more comfortable and confident. It can also help girls become more informed about their bodies and what to expect from periods.

<u>**Helpful Talking Points**</u>

When discussing periods with girls, many helpful talking points may arise. These could include topics such as menstruation, menstrual products, ovulation, and hormone regulation. It is important to address any inaccurate information they may have and correct any myths or taboos that still exist.

It can also be helpful to discuss the emotional aspects of periods, such as mood swings, energy levels, and cravings. This can help girls better understand their experiences and gain insight into how they can cope with any difficult emotions they may be feeling.

Finally, proper menstrual hygiene is an important aspect to discuss. This can include discussing the types of menstrual products available, how to properly dispose of them, and how often to change them. Additionally, it is important to discuss any dietary changes girls can make to improve their periods, such as reducing processed foods and incorporating more healthy fruits and vegetables.

It is essential to prepare yourself and girls for conversations on periods. Having the knowledge and understanding to properly address this topic can help reduce the stigma and misinformation surrounding them. Preparing yourself through research, discussing potential topics with girls, and using age-appropriate language are just some of the best practices for starting this kind of conversation. Talking about periods equips girls and women with the necessary information to understand and manage their menstrual cycles, which could ultimately improve their health and overall well-being.

# CHAPTER 2

<u>*How to Explain the Female Anatomy and Reproductive System*</u>

The female anatomy and reproductive system are complex, yet essential, aspect of a woman's body. It can be difficult to explain, especially when it comes to periods and reproduction. This chapter will provide information on the anatomy and reproductive system of women, about periods. It will explain the reproductive organs involved, and what hormones are necessary for periods to occur, and will provide a guide to explain the facts in an approachable and age-appropriate way.

<u>**Anatomy of the Female Reproductive System**</u>

When discussing the female reproductive system, it is important to understand the anatomy of the body's organs involved in the menstrual cycle. The female reproductive organs are internal, located inside the pelvis area of the body. The main organs are the vagina, uterus, ovaries, fallopian tubes, and cervix.

# The Vagina

The vagina, also known as the birth canal, is a muscular tube approximately 8-10 cm long. The vagina connects the external genitals to the inside of the body and acts as a passageway for menstrual blood, sperm, and the baby during birth.

# The Uterus

The uterus, also known as the womb, is a pear-shaped organ where a baby grows during pregnancy. The thick walls of the uterus are made up of strong muscles, which help to contract and push the baby out during childbirth.

# The Ovaries

The ovaries are 2 small, almond-shaped organs on each side of the uterus. They produce and release eggs periodically throughout a woman's menstruation cycle and also produce hormones, such as estrogen and progesterone.

# The Fallopian Tubes

The fallopian tubes are two small tubes that connect the ovaries to the uterus. They carry eggs released from the ovaries to the uterus for fertilization.

# The Cervix

The cervix is at the bottom of the uterus and opens into the vagina. It opens and closes throughout the menstrual and pregnancy cycles, to keep the uterus safe from infections and allow a baby to pass through during childbirth.

## Hormones Involved in Menstruation

The menstrual cycle is regulated by hormones, particularly two main hormones, estrogen, and progesterone. Estrogen stimulates the uterus lining to thicken for pregnancy, and when pregnancy does not happen, the lining sheds and leaves the body as menstrual flow. Progesterone is responsible for keeping the lining of the uterus thick and prevents the body from ovulating unnecessarily.

<u>**How to explain it to others**</u>

Explaining the female anatomy and reproductive system about periods and reproduction can be a challenge. It is important to provide facts in an approachable and age-appropriate manner.

When discussing the anatomy of the reproductive system and hormones with younger children, it can be helpful to use a more simplified language. It is important to explain that the uterus and ovaries are the organs responsible for making the eggs and that the hormones estrogen and progesterone are responsible for the period.

For older children, it can be beneficial to explain the anatomical features of the female body. You can explain the location of the ovaries, fallopian tubes, cervix, and uterus, how the reproductive hormones work together to influence the menstrual cycle, and what the menstrual cycle looks like. Describing the menstrual cycle in steps can help make it easier for older children to understand.

You can explain that when the female does not become pregnant, the uterus will shed its lining and this is what is released from the body as menstrual blood.

### *Conclusion*

The female anatomy and reproductive system are complex and essential aspects of a woman's body. It can be difficult to explain, especially when it comes to periods and reproduction. By understanding the anatomy of the female organs involved, and the hormones responsible for the menstrual cycle, and by providing the information in a simple and age-appropriate manner, it is possible to explain the female reproductive system and period to others. Understanding the anatomy and reproductive system of women is essential to properly care for them and maintaining their health.

# CHAPTER 3

## *How to Explain the Physical and Emotional Impact of Having a Period*

When it comes to helping girls understand the physical and emotional impact of the menstrual cycle, it is important to provide them with comprehensive, accurate, and age-appropriate information. From a young age, girls should be aware of their bodies and understand what to expect when they begin to menstruate. Preparing girls for this natural event in their lives not only makes them more comfortable during the process but also helps them to handle any physical and emotional changes that come along with it.

## Physical Impact

One of the key components of explaining the physical impact of having a period on girls is to explain what exactly menstruation is. During a girl's menstrual cycle, her uterus lining grows and thickens to prepare for the potential of pregnancy. If pregnancy does not occur, the uterus will then shed this lining as part of menstruation. Girls should be made aware that bleeding is just one of the physical signs of the menstrual cycle. Other common signs include cramps, bloating, soreness, and changes in appetite.

Girls should also be briefed on the potential risks associated with having a period. For example, girls need to be aware of the potential risk of developing infections from the use of tampons or pads. Additionally, it is important to discuss hormonal changes during the menstrual cycle that can cause headaches, mood swings, or fatigue.

It is also important to explain to girls that menstrual cycles can differ in length, amount of blood flow, and associated symptoms for different women. Some months can be uncomfortable and different from other times. It is important to be open and honest with girls about this so they can understand it is normal to have days when things are completely different.

<u>**Emotional Impact**</u>

The next part of explaining the physical and emotional impact of having a period on girls pertains to the potential emotional changes they can experience. Although emotions will vary from person to person, there are some common symptoms of pre-menstrual syndrome such as irritability, anxiety, depression, or increased sensitivity.

It is also important to stress to girls the importance of maintaining a healthy lifestyle. Eating nutritious foods, exercising regularly, and getting adequate rest can help to reduce the physical and emotional symptoms of the menstrual cycle. Additionally, girls should be made aware of activities such as yoga, meditation, and guided breathing that can help to cope with any difficult emotions they may experience.

Finally, girls should be made aware that they can always turn to a trusted adult, friend, or family member if they are not coping well with their period. It is essential that girls feel comfortable talking about their period and any associated physical or emotional changes with someone they can trust.

## *Conclusion*

Explaining the physical and emotional impact of having a period on girls is essential to helping them become comfortable with this natural event in their lives. By providing them with accurate and age-appropriate information, girls can be prepared to handle any potential changes that come along with the menstrual cycle. Additionally, it is important to stress the importance of maintaining a healthy lifestyle as well as any activities or helpful resources girls can do to cope with any associated physical or emotional changes. With adequate knowledge and awareness, girls can be better equipped to make informed decisions about their bodies.

# CHAPTER 4

*How to Explain Menstrual Period Hygiene*

Menstruation – it's a natural process that occurs with all female-identifying individuals before they reach menopause. It can be uncomfortable, and sometimes confusing and embarrassing. As such, it is important to offer children – girls in particular – the necessary awareness, knowledge, and support so that they can describe menstrual period hygiene accurately and confidently. It is vital that this education is given positively and openly – free from stigma and myths – to ensure that girls are given the support and information that they need.

By teaching girls about menstrual hygiene care, we create a more open and understanding view of menstruation in society, and better equip the next generation to talk openly and confidently about periods.

## Reasons for Menstrual Hygiene

The first step in teaching girls about menstrual hygiene is to explain the reasons for hygienic practices. Menstruation is a natural, healthy process and nothing to be ashamed of; however, it is also important to be aware of the potential risks of not being properly informed and equipped to manage it.

The most important reason for talking to girls about menstrual hygiene is to help them stay healthy. Proper menstrual hygiene helps to keep infections and illnesses away, as well as reduce unpleasant odors. Girls should be taught why it's important to keep the area clean and dry during their period and to change their sanitary products regularly, as well as to wash their hands before and after changing.

<u>**Easy to follow Steps:**</u>

One of the best ways to ensure that girls understand the importance of menstrual hygiene is to give them clear, easy-to-follow steps. Girls should be taught how to use their sanitary products correctly, cleaning and changing them regularly.

First, it is important to demonstrate how to use and dispose of sanitary products securely and with minimal mess. Girls should be taught to place used sanitary items in separate, secure bags and dispose of them responsibly.

It is also important to show girls how to wash their hands after changing sanitary products and how to shower or bathe whilst on their period, to keep the vagina clean and free from infection. Girls should be taught the importance of wearing clean, comfortable underwear and regularly changing their sanitary products, as well as washing their hands and showering regularly.

## Using Protective Products

It is also important to explain to girls the different types of sanitary products that are available, and the importance of selecting the correct one for their body shape, size, and needs. Different types of protection can be used depending on the time of the month – such as pads and tampons – and girls should also be taught how to use them correctly.

Girls should be made aware of the benefits of using protective products such as period panties and menstrual cups. It is also important to note that it is important to always use the right product for the right size and shape of the body, as well as make sure that the products are safe and comfortable.

<u>**Educating Girls**</u>

It is vital to remember that girls should be given access to accurate and reliable information regarding menstrual hygiene. Too often, misinformation is spread which is not only inaccurate but also damaging to girls' health and well-being.

Girls must be taught to question any information they hear and to look for reliable sources. Teaching girls about menstrual hygiene care is not only beneficial for their physical health, but also for promoting mental health and well-being.

Conclusion

Teaching girls about proper menstrual hygiene care is an important step in creating a positive view of periods and empowering the next generation to talk openly about the subject. Girls must be given access to accurate and reliable information regarding menstrual hygiene, as well as clear and easy-to-follow steps for managing periods.

By educating girls about menstrual hygiene, we create a more open and understanding view of menstruation in society and equip them to talk openly and confidently about periods. This not only helps to protect girls' physical health but also promotes their mental well-being.

# CHAPTER 5

## *How to Explain the Different Types of Period Products*

Period products play an important role in keeping girls comfortable and healthy during their menstruation. However, for many young girls, understanding the different types of period products available to them can seem overwhelming. As a parent, guardian, or educator, it can be helpful to understand the different period products, so you can feel more comfortable talking to young girls about them and help them to make informed decisions. In this chapter, we will discuss the various types of period products and how best to explain them to girls.

The most common types of period products used by girls today consist of pads, tampons, cups, and sponges.

# Pads

Pads are the most common type of period product used by girls, and come in a variety of sizes and absorbencies. They consist of an absorbent inner pad, covered by an adhesive, cloth-like backing to attach the pad to the user's underwear. Pads have an absorbent layer that retains menstrual fluid and are worn externally to catch and absorb menstrual flow before it reaches clothing. To use a pad, simply open the package and peel off the adhesive backing. Place the pad on the crotch of your underwear, so that the adhesive side is facing your skin. Pads can be worn for several hours, depending on flow, and should be changed multiple times per day.

# Tampons

Tampons are made up of a compact tube of soft, absorbent material. To insert a tampon, you should first unwrap it and hold it by the plunger end. Spread your legs, and place the tampon into the opening of the vagina at a 45-degree angle towards your lower back. Push the plunger of the tampon until it is comfortably inserted and the entire string is visible. To remove the tampon, simply hold the string and pull the tampon out of your vagina. Tampons should be changed every few hours, and should not be worn for more than 8 hours.

# Cups

One of the more recent innovations in period products is the menstrual cup. Menstrual cups are silicone, bell-shaped cups that are placed into the opening of the vagina. When inserted correctly, the cup forms a seal with the vaginal walls and catches and collects menstrual fluid. Menstrual cups should be emptied and rinsed every 6 to 12 hours.

# Sponges

Sponges are a type of period product that is made from absorbent cotton and is shaped like a natural sea sponge. Sponges are more absorbent than tampons and can be used in the same manner. To use a sea sponge as a period product, simply wet it with water, and insert it into the opening of the vagina. Sponges should be rinsed and changed every 4 to 6 hours.

# Explaining the Different Types of Period Products to Girls

When discussing the different types of period products for girls, it is important to discuss the advantages and disadvantages of each. Explain to girls that each type of product can work differently for each person and that, as they use each type of product, they may find that one works better for them than the others.

## Pads

Explain to girls that pads are worn externally and are attached to the underwear. Make sure that girls are aware that pads should be changed frequently to avoid feeling uncomfortable or smelly. Discuss with them the different sizes and absorbencies to help them determine which type will work best for them.

**Tampons**

Explain to girls that tampons are inserted into the vagina, and should be changed every few hours. Talk to them about how it's important to never leave a tampon in for longer than 8 hours to avoid the risk of Toxic Shock Syndrome.

**Cups**

Explain to girls that cups are not just menstrual product but a reusable device that has to be emptied and washed out every 6 to 12 hours. Tell them that cups can be a good option for girls who prefer longer-term protection.

**Sponges**

Explain to girls that sponges are slightly more absorbent than tampons and last for a few hours before needing to be replaced. Sponges can be cheaper and more environmentally friendly than other types of period products.

**Conclusion**

Menstrual products are an important part of life for many girls. It is important for them to understand the different types of period products available to them and how best to use them to stay comfortable and healthy during their menstruation. It is equally important for parents, guardians, and educators to understand the different period products and how to talk to girls about them to help them make informed decisions.

# CHAPTER 6

## *How to Discuss Stereotypes Surrounding Periods*

Stereotypes around periods have been around for a long time, and unfortunately, still exist today. Stereotypes associated with periods can make girls feel embarrassed or ashamed and can prevent them from getting the support they need or seeking out the education they deserve. Therefore, discussing stereotypes related to periods with girls is important to ensure they feel empowered and confident. This chapter provides tips and strategies for discussing period stereotypes with girls so that they understand these stereotypes are inaccurate and unfair.

## Define the Stereotype

Before you can begin discussing period stereotypes with girls, it is important to clarify what these stereotypes are exactly. Explain to them that a stereotype is an assumption about a certain type of person or group based on certain characteristics. Stereotypes about periods typically include assumptions about women's bodies, such as the notion that periods are dirty, shameful, or uncomfortably private. Stereotypes may also include the idea that periods are only experienced by women and that they are only a woman's problem.

## Explain Why Stereotypes Are Inaccurate

Once you have established what period stereotypes are, you can begin to explain why they are inaccurate. Remind girls that periods are a natural, normal part of everyone's biology and should not be discussed in a negative or demeaning way. Explain that having a period is not something to be ashamed of and it is not only experienced by women.

## Encourage Open Discussion

It is important that girls feel comfortable discussing period stereotypes and any other questions they may have about their bodies and sexuality. Encourage open discussion by letting them know it is okay to ask questions and discuss any worries or concerns they may have. Let them know that it is also okay to make mistakes and that it is perfectly normal to feel unsure or embarrassed.

## Teach Proper Terminology

Teach girls about proper terminology for anatomy and bodily functions related to periods. Girls need to be familiar with accurate terminology to make them feel more comfortable discussing the topic. Provide words and phrases that are appropriate for different ages and levels of understanding.

## Highlight Positive Role Models

Provide examples of positive role models who have publicly discussed periods and disproven stereotypes. Highlight notable figures such as celebrities, scientists, and activists who have spoken out about period shaming and the need for better period education and support. Show girls that these conversations are important and normal and that it is entirely possible to fight against period oppression and create positive change.

## Encourage Empathy

Encourage girls to be empathetic and compassionate towards each other when discussing periods. Let them know that everyone experiences periods differently and that everyone deserves to have choices and access to resources related to period care. Remind them that periods are nothing to be embarrassed about and that everyone should feel comfortable talking about and taking care of their bodies.

It is essential to talk about period stereotypes so that young girls can better understand and manage their bodies and health. This knowledge can help them make more informed decisions regarding their reproductive health. Talking openly about period stereotypes can also help them to challenge and confront these beliefs positively. It can help enhance the girls' self-image and empower them.

# How to Discuss Period Stereotypes with Girls

**1. Find the right moment**: Ask yourself if the girl is emotionally ready to talk to you about this subject. It is important to ensure that you make the conversation comfortable and tailored to the person's age and maturity.

**2. Start the conversation in a non-threatening way:** Ask the girl for her views and thoughts on the subject. This will make her feel welcomed and encouraged to talk openly about it.

**3. Show your support:** Make sure that the girl understands that you are available for her if she ever needs any help or further information.

**4. Educate and provide accurate information:** Demonstrate to the girl that menstruation is a natural process and normalizes it in her eyes. It is also important to provide her with reliable and accurate information regarding her body.

**5. Challenge negative language and attitudes:** Explain to the girl that there is nothing wrong with having a period and that it should be embraced, not shamed.

**6. Reiterate the importance of self-care:** Remind her that a positive attitude is key during her period days. Demonstrate to her that taking care of herself and eating a healthy diet can make a huge difference during this time.

Discussing stereotypes surrounding periods with girls is an important step in fostering an open, honest dialogue about periods and providing girls with the support and education they deserve. By defining these stereotypes, explaining why they are inaccurate, encouraging open discussion, teaching proper terminology, and highlighting positive role models, parents and educators can create an environment for girls to feel more confident and empowered about their bodies. Additionally, by encouraging empathy among peers, girls can ensure that everyone is being treated with respect when talking about periods and that everyone's experience is valid and appreciated.

# CHAPTER 7

## *Offering Support and Encouraging Open Questions about Periods*

As a parent or educator, it can be difficult to know how and when to talk to girls about periods. However, it is essential to discuss the topic as openly and honestly as possible to promote a culture of understanding and acceptance. Offering support and encouragement when it comes to open questions about periods can be immensely beneficial for a girl's physical, emotional and mental health, and her future well-being. This chapter offers advice on how to provide support and encouragement when talking to girls about periods and how to answer their open questions.

# 1. When to Discuss Periods and What Questions to Ask

The best time to talk to girls about periods varies by individual, but it is generally recommended to begin discussing this topic before they have their first period. The goal is to provide them with the knowledge and tools they need to feel comfortable and confident in dealing with their new body changes and period management.

Open-ended questions are the best way to begin these discussions because they allow for honest and non-judgmental dialogue that promotes informative and educational discussion. "Do you know anything about periods?" is one example of a question. "What would you like to know about periods?" and "How do you feel when you hear the word "period?". Encourage a conversation by not only asking questions but also sharing facts, stories, or anecdotes on the topic.

# 2. How to Answer Girls' Open Questions about Periods

When answering a girl's open questions about periods, it is important to do so in a factual and non-judgmental way. Avoid using words such as "icky" or "gross", which can make the girl feel ashamed of her body and its normal process. Instead, emphasize the importance and the naturalness of periods.

It's important to make sure that girls know that menstruation is a part of healthy development and to provide an accepting and understanding environment. Explain the different stages of puberty that girls go through and why hormonal changes occur. Be sure to emphasize that periods are a natural process that every woman experiences and should not be something to be embarrassed about or to feel ashamed of.

In addition, make it clear that everyone's body is different and that menstrual cycles differ from person to person. Provide information on the different products available, such as pads and tampons, and how to use them safely and hygienically.

# 3. Offering Support and Encouragement

In addition to providing factual and unbiased information, it is important to offer support and encouragement when talking to girls about periods. Emphasize that it is okay to make mistakes and that talking about periods will help them to learn and understand more about their bodies.

Remind girls that they are not alone in their experience and that there are lots of people in the same boat as them. Acknowledge that periods can be a source of stress, such as worrying about whether they are normal or if something is wrong with them.

In addition, provide tips and advice on how to manage the physical and emotional symptoms associated with periods, such as cramping, mood swings, and fatigue. Show them that you are there to help and that you understand and empathize with them.

Conclusion

Talking to girls about periods can be a daunting task. However, by providing support and encouragement and answering their open questions in an unbiased and factual way, you can help to promote an understanding and accepting environment for all women. This can lead to a healthy and positive future for generations of girls to come.

# CHAPTER 8



## *How to Explain PMS Period to Girls*

PMS, or Pre-Menstrual Syndrome, is the period of hormonal and physical changes that many girls experience in the lead-up to their menstrual cycle. Periods can be a difficult thing for teenage girls to understand, and explaining PMS to them is an important part of ensuring they are comfortable and informed about their health and bodies.

# Common Experiences of PMS

There are many experiences related to PMS that girls can expect to have. Depending on the individual, they may experience some or all of the following: Bloating, mood swings, headaches, breast tenderness, and irritability, fatigue, and food cravings. All of these symptoms can build up in the days leading up to a period and peak shortly before it starts.

# Reassuring Girls about PMS

It can be difficult for young girls to understand why they are feeling such drastic changes in their bodies and emotions. It is important to reassure them that these experiences are completely normal and part of the natural life cycle. If they have ever experienced any other physical changes, like puberty, then it can help to explain that PMS is just another process their bodies are going through as they grow up. Another way to help them understand is to simply explain that these hormonal changes are a signal that their body is preparing for the beginning of their period.

# Journaling and Keeping Track

Encourage girls to observe and keep track of their own PMS experiences. Journaling can be a great tool for them to learn about their body and the changes it goes through. They can write about their feelings, physical experiences, and how their body responds to different foods or activities - all of which can be helpful to better understand PMS. This can be a great way to build up self-confidence and help girls feel in control of their bodies.

# Managing PMS

In addition to journaling, there are a variety of things girls can do to help manage their PMS to reduce the symptoms. These include eating plenty of fresh fruit and veggies, getting enough sleep, exercising regularly, and taking breaks from stressful situations. In addition, it can be helpful to identify activities that can help reduce stress and bring back feelings of joy and relaxation, such as listening to music, reading a book, or talking to a friend.

**Conclusion**

Explaining PMS to girls is an important part of helping them understand their bodies and the changes that they go through. Reassuring them that these experiences are normal can help them feel in control, while journaling and tracking can provide valuable insight into their own experience. Finally, offering tips on how to manage their PMS can help to alleviate some of the symptoms and make the process easier to handle.

# CHAPTER 9

## *Answers to Regular Questions Asked About Periods by Girls*

### *1. What is a period?*

A period is a natural, regular part of a woman's menstrual cycle. It usually lasts between 3 and 5 days, although some women will experience a slightly longer or shorter period. During a period, the lining of the uterus—which builds up during the menstrual cycle to prepare for a potential pregnancy—breaks down and sheds, causing bleeding and the release of hormones.

### *2. What are the symptoms of a period?*

The main symptom of a period is vaginal bleeding, which can vary in amount and duration from person to person. Other symptoms may include cramps, back or abdominal pain, bloating, fatigue, headaches, breast tenderness, and mood swings.

### 3. What age do periods usually start?

Most girls get their 1st period between the ages of 10 and 16. It's normal for periods to start at any age between 8 and 15, but if you haven't had your first period by age 16, you should talk to your doctor.

### 4. Is it normal to miss a period?

It's normal to miss one or more periods, especially during puberty when hormones are fluctuating. Other reasons for missing a period include stress, illness, pregnancy, and changes in diet or exercise. If you miss two or more periods without an explanation, you should talk to your doctor.

## 5. How do I know when my period is coming?

Most women experience symptoms in the days or weeks leading up to their period. Common signs of a pending period include cramps, sore breasts, fatigue, headaches, bloating, mood swings, and increased appetite. You may also experience spotting or light bleeding in the days leading up to your period, known as "implantation bleeding."

## 6. How can I ease period cramps?

Period cramps can be quite painful, but there are several things you can do to help ease the pain. Taking ibuprofen or other over-the-counter pain medication can help, as well as taking a hot bath or shower. Other helpful measures include drinking plenty of water, exercising, and using a heating pad on your lower abdomen.

*7. How do I know when my period has stopped?*

When your period has stopped, you'll usually notice that there is no more bleeding. Some women experience spotting for a few days after the main bleeding has stopped, but this is generally a sign that the period has ended.

*8. What happens during a period?*

A period is when a female menstruates, which is the shedding of the uterine lining. This happens when a female body releases an egg, which is not fertilized by sperm. In response to this, the uterus prepares to shed its lining, which is released through the vagina as blood. This is known as a period or menstrual cycle and it typically begins in early puberty and may continue until menopause. During a period, the amount of blood released by the body can range from light spotting to heavy bleeding, with the average being around 2-3 tablespoons each cycle. During a typical cycle, most women experience mild cramping and bloating as the body works to shed its lining. Other common side effects may include irritability, mood swings, headaches, and back pain.

## 9. *How often do periods occur?*

On average, the period occurs every 28 days, although periods may come earlier or later. For some women, their periods may happen on a more irregular basis, especially during the first few years after they begin menstruating. Most women develop a better understanding of their cycle length over time.

## 10. *At what age does a period usually start?*

Most girls get their first period between the ages of 10 and 16, although it can vary greatly by individual. It is hard to predict when exactly a period will start and it can be different for everyone.

## 11. How long does a period typically last?

The length of a period can range anywhere from 2-7 days, although it's typical for it to last between 3-5 days. It is also normal for a period to be lighter or heavier in certain months depending on your hormone levels.

## 12. *What is PMS?*

PMS stands for premenstrual syndrome, and it is the name given to the physical and emotional symptoms that can occur 1-2 weeks before a period. Symptoms of PMS vary from woman to woman, but common physical symptoms include bloating, breast tenderness, headaches, and cramping. Common emotional symptoms include anxiety, irritability, mood swings, and depression. There are many treatments available for PMS, including dietary and lifestyle modifications, prescription medications, and over-the-counter medications.

## 13. *When should I seek medical help for my period?*

It is important to consult a doctor if you experience any of the following symptoms: excessive pain during your period, a period lasting longer than 7 days, missing more than 3 periods in a row, extremely heavy bleeding requiring you to change your pad or tampon more than every 2 hours, or any other symptom that is causing you significant concern

# CONCLUSION

The topic of menstruation is often a source of embarrassment, anxiety, and confusion for young girls. This is a perfectly normal thing, as it's not something we learn about in schools or discuss openly in the community. For these reasons, it can be difficult to talk to young girls about periods, let alone actually explain what they are and how it all works. The above provides helpful advice on how to explain periods to girls of any age in an effective and informative way.

Defining and Explaining the Menstrual Cycle

It is important to start by giving girls basic knowledge about the menstrual cycle and how their bodies work. Depending on their age, you can adjust the complexity of the information, but it's essential to create a basic understanding of the flow of the menstrual cycle.

The menstrual cycle is what the body does to get ready for the possibility of pregnancy. Every month the body releases an egg, which is possible to be fertilized. At the same time, the walls of the uterus build up a lining so that if the egg is fertilized, it has a place to grow and develop. If the egg is not fertilized, this lining breaks down inside the body and is released. This is what is known as a period and is a natural part of the menstrual cycle.

Explaining What to Expect During a Period

It is important also to explain what to expect during a period. This includes any physical, emotional, or mental changes and preparation for the event. This includes premenstrual symptoms, cramping, pain relief options like heat pads, and the length of time a period usually lasts.

It is important to note that periods can vary greatly from girl to girl and even from month to month. It's also important to let girls know that different products are available for periods, such as tampons, pads, and menstrual cups.

Hygiene and Body Image

Hygiene habits can also be discussed at this time. Girls should be encouraged to wear comfortable, breathable underwear and change it daily during their period. Additionally, girls should be taught that there is nothing dirty or gross about periods, which is a natural part of being a woman. It's also important to discuss body image at this time, as periods can often cause changes in the way a girl looks or feels.

Explaining periods to girls of any age can be a difficult task, but also an important one. By discussing the menstrual cycle, what to expect during a period, and hygiene and body image, girls can be better informed and more confident in their awareness. This can help reduce the embarrassment and anxiety that can surround the topic of menstruation.

www.ingramcontent.com/pod-product-compliance
Lightning Source LLC
Chambersburg PA
CBHW050824250726
48653CB00006B/2401